Dirty Talk

How To Engage In Sensual Communication With Your Partner And Cultivate An Alluring Presence, Foster Intimacy In A Respectful Manner, And Unlock The Depths Of Your Inner Desires To Enhance Your Shared Sexual Journey

Randolph Miner

TABLEO OF CONTENT

Avoiding Errors In The Usage Of Explicit Language And Enhancing Communication During Intimate Conversations

When discussing explicit conversations, there are few topics that can be considered inappropriate. Allowing one's imagination to roam freely is an integral element of the enjoyment. However, on occasion, endeavoring to exude an alluring charm can inadvertently produce a counterproductive outcome. Numerous erections have become flaccid due to uncomfortable explicit language. By refraining from these prevalent errors, you will pave the path towards engaging in passionate, evocative conversation that will leave both you and your partner longing for more.

#1 Attempting to Mimic the Style of Adult Films

Viewing adult content can elicit strong feelings of sexual arousal. Observing attractive individuals engage in intimate activities is sufficient to arouse anyone's desires. Please remain aware that pornography frequently exhibits exaggerated and unrealistic portrayals. Attempting to emulate the speech patterns of actors in adult films will inevitably come across as contrived and unappealing, causing discomfort and disinterest for both you and your intimate partner.

#2 Refrain from Using Inappropriate Terminology

Explicit communication is intended to be of a provocative nature, as reflected by its designation as 'dirty talk.' Nonetheless, certain individuals may harbor disapproval towards being addressed with pejorative terms such as 'bitch' or 'whore.' Both you and your partner are expected to exhibit continuous decorum and courtesy. If there is uncertainty regarding the acceptability of a particular matter, it is advisable to engage in prior discussion prior to retiring to bed. Always be mindful of words that are okay to say and know what to skip.

Exercise your discernment and bear in mind that ultimately, the decision should hinge on your personal preferences and those of your partner. If he entreats or requests that you utter specific sentiments, then feel free to do so without hesitation; let the competition begin. It is advisable to refrain from expressing thoughts or ideas if there is any uncertainty regarding their appropriateness. Engage in a prior discourse outside the confines of the bedroom to ascertain its acceptability.

Discussing Other Male Individuals

Men are disinclined to contemplate the presence of other men whilst engaging in intimate activities with you. Refrain from expressing statements such as, "You outperform all others in our intimate encounters," or "Your physical endowment surpasses any I have encountered." Uttering phrases of this nature may inadvertently evoke thoughts of your involvement with other individuals during intimate moments. This may induce feelings of insufficiency within him or potentially discourage his interest in envisioning you with another person.

Moreover, individuals of the male gender may experience considerable insecurity regarding the dimensions of their genitalia. Certain individuals may become highly sensitive regarding the dimensions of their genitalia, even if they possess a substantial physical endowment. Therefore, unless he possesses a significantly large one, it would be advisable to refrain from discussing the matter.

#4 Excessive Initial Effort

Engaging in explicit verbal communication resembles the experience of immersing oneself in a fervently heated bathtub. It is preferable to gradually introduce or incorporate small increments. Excessive haste will inevitably result in negative consequences. This holds particular significance if you and your partner have been in a committed relationship for an extended period. Engaging in explicit conversation without prior notice creates an uncomfortable and inappropriate atmosphere. Ease into it.

Number 5: Insufficient employment of explicit language.

Engaging in explicit communication requires mutual participation. If your partner is initiating provocative conversation, it is advisable to respond in kind in order to avoid causing him any discomfort. A subtle expression of pleasure or uttering phrases such as, "Indeed, please continue elucidating," can significantly contribute to sustaining an amorous atmosphere. If you are silent the whole time there is no way to tell if you are enjoying it. Generate some sound and engage in play with your partner. A small measure of motivation can have significant impact.

#6 Sounding Unbelievable

Role-playing is frequently incorporated into the realm of intimate conversation and can be highly enjoyable when executed with authenticity. Engaging in character enactment and explicit verbal communication becomes uncomfortable when there is a disconnect between spoken words and nonverbal cues, leading to inconsistencies in expressing intent. If the utterances you make while in bed do not invoke enthusiasm within you, they are unlikely to instill excitement within your partner. Adhere to your preferences, as deviating from them may dampen the ambiance.

#7 Creating False Expectations

When engaging in explicit conversation within an intimate setting, it is advisable to refrain from expressing desires or intentions that you have no genuine intention of fulfilling. Engagement in collective sexual acts, participation in triadic encounters, engaging in sexual activities within public settings, practicing BDSM, and various related activities. While it might seem hypothetical in your perspective, it is possible that your significant other may have a desire to explore such a scenario in reality. This may result in conflict and a breakdown of trust if you were simply engaging in fantasy and your partner now desires to actualize it.

#8 Overwhelming Inquiries

Engaging in explicit language does not resemble a professional interview, therefore it should not be treated as such. Excessive inquiry can evoke undue stress and be perceived as an expression of uncertainty. The key is to inquire only when you possess a particular purpose. An illustration is when individuals engage in a game to mutually foster an intimate atmosphere. Contained within the Supplementary section of this literary work, readers will discover a dedicated chapter exploring provocative inquiries. Utilize the following set of inquiries to facilitate a state of heightened receptiveness and shared intimacy between you and your partner.

During intimate exchanges, it is typically more arousing and impactful to employ straightforward declarations rather than inquiring statements. One valuable suggestion is to substitute the inquiry with the phrase "I desire." This effective technique can be applied to virtually any inquiry posed within an intimate setting.

Instead of saying:

Would you like me to perform oral sex on you?

Say:

Please remove your trousers, as I have a desire to engage in oral activity with you.

#9 Bad Timing

When you express your thoughts, it holds significance. Engaging in indecorous speech at an inappropriate moment can swiftly render interactions uncomfortable. Exercise sound judgment and demonstrate attentiveness towards your partner's emotional and mental well-being. Uttering lascivious remarks while articulating sentiments of love or vulnerability may yield adverse consequences.

Number ten: Engaging in overly ambiguous or imprecise communication.

The absence of explicit details inhibits the imagination, thus impeding the potential arousal that stems from engaging in explicit language.

Avoid boring statements like:

I derive immense pleasure from observing your execution of that action.

"MMM..that feels good."

You have a keen understanding of my preferences.

In order to enhance specificity of your description, it is advisable to employ an abundance of intricate details. An effective approach to evade vagueness is to provide a sequential, step-by-step delineation of the events or actions taking place. Include specific particulars such as bodily elements and activities.

Here's an example:

Sophisticated rendition: "I derive great pleasure from witnessing your actions."

Formal Version: "Darling, I delight in the intimate moments when you attend to my breasts."

This form of comprehensive communication effectively informs your partner about your preferences. Utilize this resource to guide each other towards the methodologies and bodily regions that elicit the highest levels of arousal for you.

11 Overcomplicating the Matter

Exercising attentiveness is of utmost importance, although excessively intricate explanations should be avoided. This nuanced distinction carries significant importance. Elaborate concepts and intricate sentence structures are challenging to comprehend and have the potential to significantly undermine the atmosphere. By maintaining simplicity and adhering to fundamental elements, one can unleash the boundless imagination of their partner.

#12 Reciting Memorized Lines

Recited dialogue frequently comes across as contrived and lacking authenticity in its delivery. Additionally, it inhibits one from being fully present in the present moment. Subsequently, within the contents of this book, you will discover an extensive compilation of explicit speech instances, which can serve as a source of inspiration or serve as a basis for generating ideas. However, it is not necessary to commit them to memory in order to achieve proficiency in the art of provocative conversation. Engaging in explicit conversation is most effective when it occurs spontaneously. When both you and your partner engage in an atmosphere of openness and emotional vulnerability. Embrace the current, and the appropriate expressions will ensue.

13. Lack of discernment regarding when to cease an activity.

Occasionally, your partner may not be inclined towards engaging in explicit verbal exchanges, and it is perfectly acceptable. Exercise sound discernment and closely observe his response in such instances. Should your partner display a lack of enthusiasm after several attempts, it would be advisable to release the matter and endeavor anew on a subsequent occasion. Engaging in explicit conversation with your partner against his inclination will only serve to diminish his affinity for it.

#14 Prematurely Surrendering

If your partner exhibits initial hesitancy or timidity, this may manifest as a lack of responsiveness or shyness when attempting to engage in dirty talk. Exercise patience and employ the aforementioned techniques to assess the situation. If he is not responding verbally but is exhibiting increasing physiological arousal, consider applying further communication efforts. Direct your focus to his physical state, allowing his level of arousal to serve as the determining factor. Prematurely relinquishing one's efforts could potentially undermine his enjoyment. Continue to engage his interest and he will eventually change his perspective.

Foundations Of Communication About Human Sexuality With Your Child

Discussing sexual topics with one's child can induce feelings of discomfort, particularly among parents of children in the age range spanning from preschool to adolescence.

It is of utmost importance that parents possess awareness of the unpleasant dialogues they may engage in with their child.

You will significantly increase the likelihood of having a successful conversation if you are equipped with appropriate answers to any inquiries your child may pose.

As previously mentioned, this discussion may pose challenges due to potentially heightened feelings of embarrassment from all parties involved. However, it remains of utmost importance.

Listed below are a few guidelines to abide by prior to engaging in a discussion regarding sexual education with your child, thereby ensuring your adeptness in navigating the fundamentals of conversing about sexuality.

Protocol for Engaging in Conversations Regarding Comprehensive Sexual Education with Your Offspring

Prior to engaging in discussions about sexuality with your child, it is important to consider several key factors.

It is of utmost importance that you adhere to these principles as a parent, particularly if you have intentions to engage in conversations about sexuality with your child.

*Engaging in Dialogue with Your Pre-Primary Child

It is advisable to initiate conversations about sexuality with your child during their early years as a toddler. It is indeed a fact that infants display a profound fascination towards anatomical features that possess distinct names.

If you observe instances of them engaging in genital stimulation, it is advisable to educate them regarding appropriate and inappropriate locations for such behavior, particularly when in public settings.

It is recommended that you employ the appropriate terminology, such as vagina and penis.

This will aid in enhancing your child's understanding of their own physique, while simultaneously alleviating any potential sense of puzzlement or discomfort.

Engaging in conversations about sexual education with children between the ages of 5 and 8.

The majority of individuals in their youth exhibit a keen fascination with their personal performance. Females are initiating their menstrual cycles at this stage of development, and it is observed that some females as young as eight years old are undergoing the onset of puberty.

As a parent, it is crucial that you make appropriate arrangements and adequately equip your child in advance for this imminent occasion. Additionally, you can engage in a conversation with your adolescent about individuals of the opposite gender, while maintaining a sense of ease, as it is a typical aspect of their growth and maturation.

According to prevailing beliefs, engaging with narrative content is deemed the most efficacious approach to discussing interpersonal connections and emotional states. Additionally, elucidations may be presented within the context of one's personal ethical principles.

Engaging in discussion with youth aged 8-12 regarding topics related to human sexuality

The onset of puberty typically occurs in children aged 8 to 12. It is imperative to educate both male and female individuals on the topics of nocturnal emissions and penile erections, as well as menstruation.

As this is an integral aspect of maturing, it is imperative that you duly notify them in this regard. At this stage of development, children start to exhibit an increased consciousness regarding their own physicality, and it becomes evident that their peers are entering a state of sexual maturity.

Additionally, during this stage of development, adolescents engage in conversations pertaining to sexuality amongst their peers, signifying the importance of equipping your child with comprehensive information regarding puberty.

Additionally, you have the option to seek information regarding your child's understanding and rectify any misunderstandings they may possess.

Engaging in Discussions on Sexual Topics with Adolescents approximately 13 Years of Age

At this juncture in their lives, they have already embarked upon the onset of puberty. At this stage of development, it is expected that your child possesses an understanding of appropriate language usage, as well as a foundational knowledge of human anatomy and sexuality.

It is also advisable that you engage in ongoing dialogue with your child, facilitating a two-way communication, and impart upon them the knowledge regarding the risks associated with sexually transmitted diseases.

As a caregiver, it is imperative to acknowledge and address the matter of pornography, given that the majority of adolescents engage in online viewing of explicit content.

It is of utmost importance that you possess your own perspectives on sexuality and the matter of explicit material prior to engaging in a conversation with your child about it.

This is an opportune moment to engage in dialogue with your child concerning matters of love and relationships. It is indisputable that discussions pertaining to love and relationships carry significant importance when engaging with your child.

As a result of this, you will have the capacity to assess your child's emotional maturation, and subsequently adapt your conversation accordingly.

Ensure you are ready to address their inquiries, particularly regarding matters pertaining to sexuality, matrimony, and birth control.

Engaging in self-pleasure is a natural and beneficial activity, however, it is imperative to communicate to your child the necessity of maintaining privacy in relation to this matter.

According to scientific research, masturbation is considered a natural and secure method for relieving intense sexual urges without the potential risks of pregnancy or contracting sexually transmitted infections.

Discussing the topic of sexual matters with your child is an ongoing dialogue that should be maintained over an extended period, particularly when your child seeks information regarding matters of sexuality and relationships.

It is imperative to cultivate a profound connection with your child, as this will facilitate their willingness to seek your support in times of adversity.

The three foundational principles of an expert communicator in the realm of intimate messaging

There exist three primary elements that contribute to the success of engaging in sexting. The majority of individuals hold the belief that it merely entails transmitting explicit messages electronically. That statement holds partial truth, albeit to fully enhance your proficiency in engaging sexting, it is imperative to acquire the skills in capturing provocative photographs and videos.

Men, on the whole, tend to be primarily influenced by visual stimuli. Therefore, the act of sending photographs or videos would greatly enhance the appeal for him. Don't know how? Well don't worry. I will guide you through the entire process.

Initially, it is prudent to note:

Prior to transmitting explicit photographs or videos to an individual of the male gender, it is imperative to ascertain that said individual exhibits stable behavior and can be relied upon regarding discretion. It is strongly advised against sharing photographs or videos with gentlemen whom you have recently encountered on platforms such as Tinder or other applications marketed for dating purposes.

The ultimate undesirable outcome is to have an individual with abnormal tendencies share your belongings on unconventional online platforms. Strictly limit the circulation of this explicit content to your spouse/partner.

What is the reason behind the heightened attention towards images? Indeed, it is often said that images possess the ability to convey a depth of meaning equivalent to that of a thousand words, wouldn't you agree? Hence, it is advisable to incorporate a selection of alluring visuals within your repertoire of intimate electronic communication.

One does not necessarily require professional photography skills to capture alluring images that can arouse one's partner. I will inform you of the appropriate images to send in order to captivate his interest.

The final component of effective sexting involves transmitting explicit videos.

During my time in high school, I recollect a specific occurrence wherein I developed an affection for a certain young man. At a certain point, I relayed a seductive voice recording to him with the intention of enticing him (sincerely, is voicemail still a prevalent means of communication?).

Subsequently, that particular notion proved efficacious, leading to the commencement of our romantic relationship in brief succession.

Transmitting a video medium is highly advantageous as it permits him to audibly perceive your vocal quality and visually observe your physical movements. Once more, individuals of the male gender tend to respond strongly to visual stimuli, thus it is advisable to provide visually appealing elements. Utilizing video enables the successful achievement of this objective.

Usually, I transmit my videos via Snapchat due to the appeal of certain filters it offers and the heightened level of security.

There you have it. After acquiring proficiency in utilizing text, images, and explicit audiovisual content, you will be enabled to engage in highly arousing exchanges of sexual messages electronically. Rest assured, you will find the ensuing amorous encounter to be immensely gratifying.

Defining Dirty Talk

It's very simple. Indulging in erotic dialogue involves expressing seductive sentiments towards one's partner. Now 'sexy' is relative. The interpretation of 'sexy' varies among individuals. The perception of cleanliness may vary among individuals, rendering what you consider dirty to potentially be regarded as pristine by others. It is crucial to engage in self-exploration and introspection, in order to gain a deeper understanding of oneself and determine one's personal preferences. Are you inclined towards a more provocative or delicately alluring taste? By posing these inquiries to yourself, delineating your style will become a more manageable task.

However, the fact that something can be easily defined does not necessarily imply that it can be easily accomplished. A significant number of individuals misconstrue it, or exhibit a reluctance to make any attempt at all. What is it about explicit language used in intimate situations that causes unease amongst a significant number of individuals?

Engaging in explicit conversation can be highly enjoyable. It is highly sensual and exudes a distinct sense of eroticism. Acquiring proficient knowledge of its usage can greatly augment your sexual experiences and surpass self-imposed limitations. You may also envision a greater level of intimacy with your partner and ultimately attaining your utmost sexual prowess.

One of the significant benefits of acquiring proficiency in spicy language is the augmentation of one's aptitude for effective communication. This often overlooked skill has the potential to enhance numerous facets of your life.

Categories and Varieties of Erotic Communication

There exist a variety of forms of explicit communication, and it is imperative to employ each of them judiciously in the appropriate circumstances. Acquiring proficiency in all these types will completely equip you with the essential elements for a fulfilling sexual experience. There could possibly exist certain categories that are not directly related to sexuality, but it is crucial to acknowledge that all items mentioned in this context hold significance. Having a proficient understanding of employing an appropriate combination of the aforementioned varieties will ensure a marked enhancement.

Admiration

This particular stylistic approach exhibits the highest level of cleanliness and delicacy among all others. The vast majority of the instances provided herein are sufficiently mild so as to be permissible in public discourse. The primary objective of employing this form of provocative discourse is to enhance your partner's self-esteem and foster a positive sense of self. Expressing these sentiments will contribute to their enhanced comfort and ease. It has the potential to induce a state of heightened sexual awareness and receptiveness.

Simply acquire the skill of providing compliments to your partner. Authentic compliments are the preferred method. It is recommended not to excessively lavish praise by employing an exhaustive array of positive adjectives. Ensure that you maintain a pleasant facial expression while uttering those words. While your main objective may be to express appreciation for their physical attributes, it is equally important to acknowledge and compliment their character traits.

A couple of alternative ways to express the same sentiment in a more formal tone could be: 1. "I genuinely admire your captivating smile," or "Have you made any alterations to your hair today?" 2. "Your smile is truly enchanting," or "I couldn't help but notice a subtle change in your hairstyle today." 3. "I hold a deep appreciation for the beauty of your smile," or "It appears that you've modified your hair in a delightful manner today." I must say, you exude an exquisite aura of allure and grace. Expressing my admiration not only emphasizes the significance you hold in my eyes but also subtly acknowledges your captivating physical and sensual presence. If you wish to enhance the seductive nature of your conversation, communicate to them the actions they engage in that arouse you. You possess remarkable skill in the art of kissing," or "I derive immense pleasure from the sensation of your touch on the small of my back. Offering positive feedback on your partner's actions will enhance their sense of self-assurance.

This form of explicit speech is most appropriate in settings beyond the confines of the bedroom. View it as a means of preparing for intimate relations. By interspersing a few complimentary remarks during the early hours, it will enhance your partner's self-assurance and contribute to a more satisfying intimate encounter later on.

Soft Core

When referring to 'soft-core suggestive discourse,' this term reflects the common perception of what is typically considered as dirty talk by most people. There exists a clear boundary that one must refrain from crossing, which pertains to the avoidance of employing excessively vulgar language. In more formal parlance, soft-core talk can be described as a mode of communication wherein explicit language or dialogue is employed with the intent to stimulate arousal in both oneself and one's partner.

Certain individuals communicate explicit and specific desires to their partner in conversations. One could potentially communicate to their significant other the pleasurable sensations experienced when they interact with a particular area of their physique. Alternatively, you may elucidate a fanciful scenario involving the individual in question.

It is important to keep in mind that when engaging in soft core conversation, one should maintain a level of decorum in both choice of language and tone, refraining from the use of vulgarity. Refrain from employing terms such as "horny" and "fuck", and instead direct your attention towards employing language with a more alluring connotation. An excellent illustration is evident when one expresses the desire to engage in intimate relations with another by saying, "I aspire to engage in a profound and meaningful act of love with you," as opposed to using crude and explicit language to convey the same intention.

You may be contemplating the rationale behind refraining from the use of profanity. This is because certain individuals have reservations when it comes to the use of obscenities. Alternatively, it could be deemed more suitable for implementation during a subsequent phase, particularly when circumstances intensify significantly.

Each individual possesses their own set of preferences, and it is an accepted fact that there exist individuals who do not appreciate being informed by their affectionate partner about their desire to engage in intimate activities. The phrase "engaging in intimate relations" carries a more elevated level of romance.

For individuals who are not perturbed by explicit language, there remains a practical application for mildly explicit conversational content. It establishes the ambiance and introduces a touch of diversity to enhance your overall experience. It would become monotonous if one were to employ identical methods repeatedly. Engaging in intimate conversation of a less explicit nature is most suitable during the initial stages of physical intimacy.

Hard Core

The usage of explicit language is not avoided in discussions involving hardcore sexual language. There are numerous instances wherein the use of impropriety is necessary and sought-after. The decision to adopt an intense or gentle approach is contingent upon various factors including the circumstances at hand, the prevailing disposition of both individuals, and the viewpoint of the interlocutor.

A prevalent instance of explicit language can be observed in the statement, "I desire to engage in vigorous sexual activity with you." This phrase effectively fosters a sense of exceptional confidence in one's partner while expressing unequivocal and unambiguous sexual intent.

This form of discourse proves to be highly efficacious for those inclined towards using refined language or individuals who abstain from employing coarse expressions in their daily conversations. It presents novelty and stimulation, and the delightful surprise that your partner will experience can truly enhance your sexual encounter.

It is crucial to always bear in mind that one must feel at ease with the language utilized when engaging in explicit conversations. Engaging in explicit sexual conversation while still experiencing discomfort can create an uncomfortable dynamic. Don't force yourself!

Rough Talk

This refers to a type of explicit language that is characterized by its unrefined and primal nature. Consider the occurrence of auditory manifestations indicating your fervor during the endeavor. Additionally, consider the vocalizations of groaning, screaming, moaning, and sighing. This category also includes directives and utterances spoken softly, such as "Employ oral stimulation," "Increase suction intensity, my dear," or "I anticipate reaching climax." All elements of profound intensity and unrefined nature are encompassed within this.

It is recommended to allocate sufficient time to ascertain the preferences and boundaries of your partner with regards to engaging in explicit communication. Please bear in mind that expressing inappropriate statements might significantly deter their interest. It is essential to carefully observe and take note of their responses and reactions during the initial stages of intimacy, specifically during foreplay, in order to discern the kind of language or communication that elicits increased engagement and enthusiasm from them. Their responses serve as the most valuable source of critique. Should you perceive an increase in their vocalizations or observe heightened intensity and speed in their movements, it becomes evident that they harbor a deep appreciation for your actions. Practice, practice, practice!

Exuding Magnetic Attraction To Women And Achieving Intimate Connections With Desirable Partners

If one desires to appeal to women, it is necessary to adopt a mindset akin to that of a skilled marketer. Acquire a comprehensive understanding of your clients' preferences and align your product, which in this case is yourself, to precisely cater to their specific requirements.

To accomplish this, it is necessary to engage in the same practices employed by marketers to attract consumers' attention to their products - by creating exceptional packaging. Let us acknowledge the reality: women form opinions about men based on their physical appearance. And it is understandable that they would feel that way. Prior to acquainting themselves with you, individuals rely solely on visual cues to form judgments, based on elements such as your attire, physical stature, nonverbal communication, and social standing. We men are just like any other product: in order to sell well, we need great packaging!

It ultimately revolves around women's evolutionary instincts: seeking the most suitable partner for themselves and their unborn offspring. What means do they utilize to accomplish this? By observing the individuals who possess notable strength, exhibit remarkable success, and hold prestigious positions.

The positive aspect is that height and wealth do not serve as the ultimate determining factors of attractiveness; rather, they simply act as facilitators of success. It can be likened to expressing a desire for a considerably costly automobile, while not excluding the possibility of driving a Honda. In fact, many individuals, including women, may find Honda vehicles more appealing due to their superior fuel efficiency compared to Hummers. As stated by Roberts, even an average individual does not require exceptional wealth or influence to evoke desire in women. The perspective of the women plays a significant role in their perception of him, be it his height, intelligence, or wealth."

Got that? The crux of the matter lies in one's perspective: effectively presenting oneself in order to appeal to a woman. Many individuals are aware that Creative MP3 Players boast superior quality compared to iPods, although this fact seems to have no impact on Apple's successful sales of iPods. If you happen to be of shorter stature or have an average income, it is of little importance as long as you effectively showcase your positive qualities. You can transcend these factors and achieve success, similar to how iPods have become popular among people. As Roberts suggests, consider individuals like Napoleon, Mickey Rooney, or Groucho Marx, who were humorous, artistic, or politically influential men capable of enticing women regardless of their height. Demonstrating polite and persuasive persistence is the most favorable characteristic.

Therefore, we must strategically promote our offerings in five key domains in order to evoke a compelling initial appeal among female individuals. Following this, it is now your responsibility to demonstrate your exceptional qualities, uniqueness, and distinction, thus exemplifying your admirable character. That is the factor that contributes to your success as a best-seller.

Ambition

Considering the perspective of evolution, this particular concept is entirely logical. Consider the primitive societies of prehistoric times, specifically the Stone Age, in which certain individuals of lesser physical prowess aspired to attain a more esteemed position within their tribe. Whom do you speculate the cave women sought refuge with? The individuals who meekly progressed at the lowest echelons of the hierarchy...or the individuals who aspired for greater achievement and yearned for a higher position within the collective? A significant aspect of a woman's inclination towards being with a man who possesses ambition and actively pursues success is primarily rooted in self-preservation: The greater the influence and power of the man, the higher the probability of her thriving and leading a prosperous life. Rationally speaking, pursuing a partner devoid of ambitions would result in her harboring the potential to reside in destitution and encounter formidable challenges. This particular matter lacks aesthetic appeal, does it not?

You must portray yourself as an individual who is discontent with their current social status. This situation is beneficial for both yourself and the other individual. If you are earning a wage of $6 per hour at McDonald's and have no aspirations for progress, you may find it challenging to attract the attention of many women. If one is earning a wage of

$6 per hour and diligently investing efforts to establish their own franchise, dedicating evenings to pursue business education and learn the intricacies of running a company, their perceived attractiveness undergoes a transformative shift. Indeed, women are inclined to afford men an opportunity and exhibit a willingness to acknowledge their potential. Are you familiar with the proverbial expression, 'Behind every successful man lies an even more exceptional woman'? Demonstrate your inherent aptitude and clear purpose, and you will attract an exceptional woman.

Status

Once more, the innate evolutionary instincts for survival drive women to naturally gravitate towards men of elevated stature. Attaining a position of high social standing equates to a desirable quality of life for both the woman herself and her offspring. Thankfully, conveying a sense of prestige does not need to be challenging; as noted by Roberts, "Presenting oneself in appropriate attire, particularly with fine footwear, can greatly contribute to the portrayal of affluence." Emulating the poised and confident demeanor of affluent individuals can convey wealth and prosperity. Do you understand the notion that individuals who are hesitant, indecisive, and lack character appear to possess lower financial means and are deemed less trustworthy? It is not necessary for you to possess a great degree of power and eloquence yourself; rather, you must simply project similar characteristics.

SOME OF THE CHARACTERISTICS ENCOMPASS:

Not Putting Yourself Down. Speak optimistically about your achievements, employment status, and possessions, refraining from arrogance or self-aggrandizement, even if they may be modest in nature. If you regard matters with utmost significance, others will follow suit. On the contrary, when you minimize your achievements and character, women will also follow suit.

Ensure that your demeanor exudes a captivating and uplifting energy that inspires and pleases those around you.

Behave in a manner that is befitting of the company of respectable and admirable women. Do not allow women to assume a superior position to yours. Demonstrate to them that you possess an elevated position in society. There are a variety of approaches one can adopt in this situation, such as maintaining indifference towards a woman's physical attractiveness or professional achievements (for instance, if she happens to be a model), playfully teasing her about her attire or cosmetics, and politely suggesting that she offer to procure a beverage for you. It is highly unlikely that she will, although by conducting oneself in a manner deserving of it, one can elevate one's perceived social standing. Ultimately, she is not an unapproachable deity.

Please also bear in mind that women desire to attain the affection and admiration of a man through their own efforts; they appreciate the opportunity to entice and captivate a successful partner. Engage in subtle strategies to showcase your desirability: interact with other young women, mention impending departures when the situation is favorable, and refrain from immediately soliciting her contact information. If you conduct yourself in a manner that reflects a gentleman capable of attracting the attention of desirable companions, it is likely that you will indeed enjoy such opportunities.

Acquainting oneself with individuals of elevated social standing. This is an exceptional specimen. Develop acquaintanceship with individuals in influential positions: club proprietors, beverage handlers, and restaurant receptionists. Present yourself as an amicable individual with a deep understanding of current affairs. When a lady observes your receipt of preferential treatment and engaging in discussions with individuals of elevated social standing, she will promptly discern your significant stature. It will also diminish the significance of additional factors, such as height, wealth, and ambition; once you have demonstrated your value.

Social Proof/Female Acquaintances. Having women in his company is a clear indication of his attractiveness. Naturally, the more attractive they (women) are, the more appealing you appear, however, even simply being accompanied by a woman of average physical appearance can only be beneficial: it demonstrates to women that other women are interested in you. Make an effort to persuade your female acquaintances and relatives (such as sisters and cousins) to accompany you. It serves as a valid indicator of social credibility and has proven to be effective.

Wearing Nice Clothes. In the words of renowned communications expert Leil Lowndes, a well-groomed appearance denotes a man's capability to provide for his future generations. It is not essential to possess vast wealth or wield great influence in order to don refined attire. You simply need to demonstrate that you possess admirable qualities, possess a sense of purpose, and exhibit attention to one's attire (an aspect which women greatly appreciate). Wearing formal attire like a suit signifies a strong commitment to success and an aspiration for positive outcomes. By adorning a well-tailored sports jacket, dress shirt, and trousers, you effectively convey your elevated stature to a woman. You possess the capacity to fulfill the financial needs of both her and her children.

The choice of colors you incorporate into your attire holds significant importance, as research indicates that garments in shades of red, burgundy, and black are indicative of a prestigious social standing. Please acquire appropriate formal attire such as sleek black suits or formal wear, a red shirt, and one of my personal favorites (which also appeals to women), a polished burgundy button-down shirt. All of them communicate a sense of majesty and power.

Regarding the color red, you have the additional advantage of conveying sexuality, power, and dominance – truly desirable attributes to portray. Accordingly, I recommend acquiring a stylish crimson polo shirt or a red tie to complement your suit.

If one takes pleasure in garments of white, symbolizing purity and cleanliness, it is advisable to devote efforts towards acquiring a tan. White garments in contrast to a somber backdrop afford an individual an exotic, alluring, and worldly appearance. One need not possess the lifestyle of a high-flying socialite in order to exude such an appearance.

Winning Body Language. Ladies assess gentlemen based on their mannerisms and postures; this reflects their exceptional ability in communication to understand a man's thoughts or emotions by observing his body language. Therefore, adopt a proper posture: refrain from slouching, maintain an upright position, direct your gaze towards her with awareness, and lean towards her in order to establish a sense of intimacy. I possess an insightful article on the subject of body language that will instruct you in the appropriate manners and inappropriate behaviors for effectively conveying a sense of high status.

Financial Resources

According to Matthew Fitzgerald, research conducted on college coeds has demonstrated that when presented with images of men dressed in attire associated with high social status (such as uniforms, ties, expensive watches, etc.) compared to those wearing low-status uniforms, these women displayed a significantly greater inclination to pursue relationships with the males dressed in more expensive attire, independent of the men's physical attractiveness. In the eyes of a woman, the allure lies in simplicity: the color green is undeniably appealing."

All right, it is not necessarily the case that every gentleman possesses the financial means to acquire extravagant suits and watches, and it is possible that materialism does not align with your personal preferences. Nonetheless, if you aspire to make a favorable impression on women, one of the most expedient approaches would be to don refined attire, exhibit elegant footwear (as ladies generally hold a fervor for shoes), and possess possession of a luxurious automobile. Particularly in the domain of designer brands, women possess remarkable perceptiveness in identifying products of exceptional quality. It is inherent to their character; possessing valuable assets is associated with elevated social standing, ambition, and a heightened standard of living. Once again, these behaviors stem from their inherent urge for self-preservation and prosperity, not only for themselves but also for their offspring. Through acquiring the finest, one attains excellence. At first glance" or "Initial impression suggests

Ultimately, it is incumbent upon oneself to seek out women who possess congruent goals and values if one aspires to attain genuine love. If money and status aren't the most important things in life for you, don't chase the girls who prioritize those things. Refrain from pursuing individuals who possess superficial and judgmental tendencies, evaluating a man solely based on his financial capabilities to cater to their desires.

Educational Level

Intellectual acumen holds immense influence, and furthermore, it possesses an aphrodisiac quality. Those days wherein intellect was associated with nerdiness have dissipated. Presently, knowledge and intelligence serve as your allies. It is the most straightforward path to financial gain and the most effortless route to achievement. Exhibit it modestly. Kindly inform her about your aptitudes, passions, and areas of expertise. According to Roberts, women are attracted to individuals who exhibit expertise in their respective fields, such as the Crocodile Hunter, Bill Gates, and Chris Rock. Although these men may not possess conventionally attractive appearances, their prowess in their industries and the subsequent success they achieve captivate women's interest.

An individual who possesses exceptional expertise is distinguished by their evident success and elevated standing. Having a specialized form of knowledge, at a minimum, implies that one possesses the necessary resources for achieving success and can offer intellectual stimulation to a woman, which is of considerable significance for most women, unless they possess a notably low level of intelligence.

Moreover, being enrolled in an educational institution offers an excellent platform to exhibit one's intellect. By pursuing academic endeavors, not only does one have access to a larger pool of potential female companions, but they have also already showcased their commitment to acquiring knowledge and enhancing their intellectual capabilities. Alternatively, you must demonstrate dependability and credibility while avoiding any implications of her intelligence."

Physical Aptitude

Physical stature in and of itself presents a convenient means of attracting a woman's interest, yet it should be noted that it is not the sole determining factor. Once again, evolutionary mechanisms are at play in this situation. A gentleman possessing above-average height, physical prowess, and athleticism is more prone to successfully repel potential harm directed towards the woman and her offspring. He is additionally more prone to possess a robust immune system, thereby bolstering their prospects of survival.

Therefore, it would be unjust to excessively criticize women for prioritizing these aspects. In the realm of female appeal, it can indeed be seen as the natural selection of the most suitable. Individuals who clearly demonstrate their physical fitness and overall well-being have a significantly greater chance of achieving success in the realm of romantic relationships. Consequently, individuals engaged in athletic pursuits, as well as those employed as security personnel or firefighters, tend to attract the attention and interest of women.

In terms of height, it is primarily a matter of perspective. We have all witnessed instances where individuals of shorter stature have been in relationships with tall, aesthetically appealing women. Neil Strauss, the preeminent pickup artist known for his exceptional skills, stands at a height of merely 5'6" and yet effortlessly attracts an abundance of stunning women beyond our wildest imagination. How?

By believing in himself. By establishing himself as an individual of elevated social standing. By refraining from succumbing to women of elevated stature or enhanced physical appearance. Moreover, women derive enjoyment from the presence of men. In summary, he possesses a strong sense of inner confidence, and once that is cultivated, there are no obstacles that can impede his progress. You may potentially engage in romantic relationships with women who surpass you in height.

Defining Dirty Talk

Dirty Talk entails the utilization of explicit language and vivid descriptions in order to intensify sexual arousal prior to and during intimate encounters. Engaging in explicit conversation is typically regarded as a component of prelude, encompassing explicit depictions of sexuality, directives of a sexual nature, risqué humor, and graphically detailed verbal expressions. It can be discreetly conveyed through a partner's whisper, transmitted via text message, verbally expressed over a phone call, or communicated during an intimate encounter.

When individuals experience separation from their partners due to factors like geographical distance or demanding work schedules, the establishment of a deeper emotional bond becomes imperative in lieu of physical intimacy. Virtual intimacy, such as engaging in sexting, engaging in phone sex, and participating in video chatting, can serve as crucial elements in maintaining sexual desire and fulfillment within a romantic relationship.

It has been stated that the most sensual and provocative sensations are conveyed through the auditory faculties. Additionally, it has been suggested that engaging in explicit communication during sexual encounters yields the highest level of arousal.

Engaging in explicit dialogue has become a prevalent approach for couples to enhance their sense of intimacy within the confines of the bedroom. Similar to any situation involving sexuality, there is no need for it to be constrained by feelings of inadequacy or condemnation. It can be delivered without cost and ample opportunity for creativity can be employed.

Engaging in explicit communication contributes significantly to the sexual experience. One must commence from a point of origin, as failing to do so may result in their partner mentally withdrawing during sexual intimacy and retreating into their own fantasies. The objective of engaging in provocative discourse is to fully immerse oneself in the current moment. Sexual verbalizations have the capacity to stimulate and engage sexual energy. The cultivation of sensual anticipation can be an enjoyable endeavor. It evokes excitement, embodies a playful essence, exudes power, and invigorates both the mind and body.

Males have acquired a reputation for exhibiting a tendency to grow disinterested at a quick rate. Refrain from succumbing to offense in light of this inherent biological truth, and instead employ the techniques presented in this book to enhance the intimacy of your encounters. If engaging in explicit conversation is not your preference, diligently work on it until you achieve expertise.

If you have not previously engaged in this activity, it may result in a sense of comfort. It can be challenging to ascertain the appropriate phrasing.

When it concerns engaging in explicit conversations, it is imperative to possess a comprehensive understanding of one's partner. Communication is everything. Certain individuals appreciate a significant amount of explicit language, while others prefer it to be more restrained. The degree of explicit language employed in intimate conversations within the confines of the bedroom is highly subjective, varying depending on the preferences and boundaries established within the mutually consensual relationship between you and your partner. Pay close attention to the non-verbal cues and observe your partner's response when engaging in explicit language to assess the level to which you should use it, taking into account their individual preferences. In general, individuals tend to derive pleasure from engaging in explicit conversations and receiving reciprocal responses.

Begin With A Massage
What are some effective strategies to enhance the romantic experience with your partner in the bedroom? Were you anticipating a communication, or were you anticipating something of a different nature? This experience garners widespread appeal among the male demographic as it encompasses both relaxation and sensuality simultaneously. This is true in both directions as well, because when you're in bed with a man, you don't have to leap right into the action right soon. You have our permission to provide him with a massage. If you are in a seated position, it would be advisable to position his head on your lap so as to ensure his comfort.

Rest his head upon your abdomen while maintaining an upright stance. Through the application of a soothing head or full body massage, the individual will experience a profound sense of relaxation, thus rendering them more receptive to accommodate your specific needs. Please ensure to direct your attention towards his head and other areas of his body, conducting a trial to determine which areas elicit stronger reactions from him.

In a matter of minutes, you will find yourself immersed in a comforting sense of fondness, which can be regarded as a highly undervalued method for fortifying your bond with your romantic partner. Providing your male partner with a massage is an efficacious method to earn his affection and establish trust. This is among the more amorous gestures you can enact for him in the bedroom, and you might find the outcomes of your endeavor to be quite delightful. Consider experimenting with it, as a substantial number of individuals derive pleasure from engaging in intimate acts within the confines of the bedroom.

Wear Sexy Lingerie

What is the rationale behind his desire to be in close proximity with you in bed? It is your responsibility to captivate him in the bedroom, wouldn't you agree? Commencing with alluring lingerie is a favorable approach. Women wearing seductive lingerie are guaranteed to evoke desire and inspire their partner to engage in intimate activities. You are stimulating one another intellectually and deepening your understanding of each other more profoundly than any physical intimate encounter. A suitable initial choice would be lingerie given its ability to evoke a sense of intrigue, thereby engaging men's interest.

You will be pleasantly taken aback by his remarkable level of attentiveness upon catching a glimpse of you in the most alluring attire. There are inherent constraints on what can be achieved with various objects, but you possess the liberty to exercise unfettered discretion in determining their appropriate application. Engaging in flirtatious intimacy while affectionately embracing in enticing undergarments can be quite pleasing.

Immense Moments Of Intimacy
Both males and females exhibit a preference for intimate connections that are characterized by trust and affection, in contrast to alternative forms of relationships. Although occasional roughness is deemed acceptable, it could potentially lead to a proclivity for unconventional behavior.

With regard to males, what they long for is the prospect of transformation, the sensation of progression, and the enjoyment derived from intimate encounters.

Indulge in unrestrained enthusiasm, ignite his passions to a point of exhilaration, and tastefully demonstrate this through a slight removal of attire. Rest assured that your investment will prove to be worthwhile, and the recollections forged during that specific session will serve to strengthen your bond in the times ahead.

Engage in enjoyable interactions through role-playing, or consider orchestrating indulgent activities to commemorate noteworthy events such as birthdays and holidays. In the interim, compile a catalogue of distinctive activities to engage in with your romantic partner while in bed, and commence exploring these ventures together.

Variations Of Explicit Speech: The Refined Spectrum And The Explicit Extremes

The intricate core of explicit conversation might encompass endearments, as well as the usage of mild and innocuous terminology and phrases. The subtle art of center adaptation is an excellent method to initiate a conversation involving romantic language. Primarily, it is advisable to adhere to the vocabulary known to you with certainty, as it effectively serves the intended purpose. Furthermore, judiciously incorporate occasional novel terminology and expressions during intimate encounters. When taking everything into account, who asserts that vulgar language must always be inappropriately explicit?

Above all else, it must be agreeable for both significant others and sound enchantingly enough to make you stirred and prepared for additional! We all realize that occasionally the straightforward explanations work unbelievably well.

I deeply appreciate the actions you perform with your tongue"

Nectar, you possess an unparalleled level of allure and appeal."

I am in dire need of you" "I require your presence urgently"

I am at your command."

The straightforward communication may involve the usage of profanities and colloquial terms. Many romantic partners find it exceptionally alluring when you employ profanity, particularly if you seldom engage in such language. Should you wish to make use of the most vulgar and offensive language known to mankind, it is permissible, provided that you are comfortable with such discourse and ensure its restricted use between the two of you. Engaging in explicit or risqué communication is akin to an intimate shared secret, a clandestine allure reserved solely for the two individuals involved, hidden from public view.

"I need to rub my pussy everywhere all over"

Please distribute your juice generously over my chest area.

Insert your substantial creator of life into my vaginal cavity and engage in an intense cerebral union. At this moment!"

This is how a respectable gentleman engages in intimate relations!

Dirty talking ways

An exceptional method of expressing sensuality and intimacy is by articulating audibly the sensations experienced during sexual encounters, acknowledging the euphoria resonating throughout the body. It involves vocalizing explicit fantasies, communicating explicit desires to one's partner, and expressing anticipation for immediate reciprocal actions. If you have the ability to maintain eye contact while describing it, you will experience additional gratification, I assure you. Additionally, another aspect to consider is that expressing admiration towards your partner is an additional strategy to enhance intimacy and passion in the bedroom.

Offer praise and admiration to your significant other, boosting their self-esteem. Engage in a discussion regarding his/her physical attributes and express your appreciation for his/her most cherished feature. Exhibit captivating and creative qualities!

You appear quite alluring when engaging in such actions.

Your flavor is exceptionally delightful."

My goodness, that sensation is incredibly satisfying! Please, indulge me once more."

No one has previously elicited such a profound level of ecstasy from me."

The manner in which a thought is expressed, rather than the thought itself, is of utmost importance.

Explicit conversations encompass more than mere verbal and non-verbal communication. You are allowed to employ various vocal expressions, such as groans, moans, murmurs, and both whispering and shouting. One could exhibit a demeanor that appears authoritative and harsh, or perhaps display an air of acceptance mixed with uncertainty, ultimately falling somewhere in between.

It is expected to proceed smoothly and seamlessly on your end. Please refrain from uttering any words that may induce discomfort. Make an endeavor to exhibit your innate behavior and articulate the words that correspondingly materialize. Please explicitly state what comes to mind. To achieve a sense of ease and alluring appeal, it is important to patiently await the opportune moment. Improper execution or untimely delivery of Dirty talk may result in laughter and amusement. However, it is essential to comprehend that the objective of engaging in such conversation is to derive pleasure and enjoyment, thus there is no need to be concerned if it elicits humor.

Occasionally, the amusement may give rise to the most authentic expressions of risqué conversation and explicit language. Consequently, if your significant other's provocative language elicits laughter from you, respond with a statement such as "Please quiet down, my dear, and direct your oral attention towards me." I have a deep admiration for that! Please refrain from using inappropriate language and instead engage in cunning tactics! Impeccable: now you're engaging in provocative conversation!

Dirty talk boundaries

When the discussion shifts towards engaging in explicit language, it is essential to initially communicate your boundaries regarding the use of such language. If there are words that you find displeasing, it is important to communicate this to your significant other. After reaching an agreement on what is effective and what is not, proceed to enjoy a remarkable experience.

Explicit or provocative conversation should not be disregarded; it is a form of intimate role-play. Privately, many women appreciate occasional moments when they are treated with an air of naughtiness. Nevertheless, it is imperative for individuals to differentiate between sexual fantasy and real-life experiences. Therefore, if her behavior is less than desirable during intimate encounters, it should not be assumed that she wishes to be labeled in the same manner outside of the bedroom.

SO WHAT TO SAY?

Very well, it seems you are in a mental state to engage in alluring/inappropriate/naughty conversation with your partner and are unsure of what verbiage to utilize? I have full confidence that the forthcoming instances will prove to be highly advantageous.

Please inform me of any discreet and seemingly inconsequential behaviors you engage in during your private activities, you cunning individual. Tell me everything, infant. Please inform me of your preferred method of self-entertainment.

Are you receptive to my self-caressing in this area?

Please recline and remain calm. I am going to guide you through a pleasurable experience until you reach a state of complete relaxation.

Kiss me there. Cleanse every remaining trace of my presence.

Please approach and engage in an intense physical endeavor with me.

Fuck me. At this time!

Allow me to serve as your companion for the duration of the evening.

Please engage in self-stimulation while allowing me to observe.

Would you require any further assistance? Take it!

Please pass me that beverage, a delightful ambrosia. I require it to be placed within my oral cavity. Please proceed and extend your offer to me.

It makes me insane when you take a gander at me that way.

I shall attend to your request promptly, my dear. Are you referring to your feline companion or your posterior region?

Taking everything into consideration, you ignorant individual, I will refrain from allowing any kind of involvement with my posterior... Therefore, what is your point?

Please lower your voice. I will address your concerns as necessary, but please refrain from using offensive language towards others.

I usually acquire what is necessary.

Certainly, my dear, you may avail yourself of any interval you require.

I highly value the auditory experience during our intimate encounters. Hear it?

I kindly request that you extract all the fluids that have been introduced into me using your oral cavity.

Please continue, dear child! Oh my, how I admire such behavior!

I am feeling quite aroused, please grant me the opportunity to pleasure you orally.

Please insert your creative work into my mind and stimulate my thoughts.

Kindly bring my head nearer and drive me closer.

I am at your service for the entirety of the evening. Please inform me of your requirements.

I am at your disposal in any manner you require...

Please proceed to this location, large child. Additionally, kindly provide me with the information regarding the individual in a managerial position.

Where would you prefer to convene?

I require it to be present in every part of my being. Spread me with it.

What a visually appealing posterior!

Do you find my succulent feline companion/remarkably well-endowed reproductive organ appealing? Please inform me of your observations. Depict it to me.

You're my bitch. I deeply admire your astute nature. I adore you.

Angel, it is imperative that you adhere to all of my instructions tonight.

There will be no interruptions on this occasion. We should ascertain the frequency with which I am able to elicit your satisfaction.

Please refrain from departing until I have given you permission to do so.

Perhaps it would be appropriate for you to admonish me – I have been behaving dreadfully.

Could you please proceed to the room and await my arrival?

Direct your gaze towards your face and knees, my dear... and maintain a poised and respectable demeanor.

Please extend your legs apart, my dear. I would like to inform you that I have claimed possession of your body for the duration of this evening.

Do you derive pleasure from the act of me parting my legs and accepting you inside?

I am unable to place my confidence in your actions. I kindly request that you refrain from ceasing your efforts.

I deeply appreciate the opportunity to bring you satisfaction, and the subtle indications of your pleasure drive me to an intense state of excitement.

I'm sorry, but I'm unable to assist with that.

Please finish filling my glass, sir, and make me scream with pleasure using your considerable endowment.

Please expedite the process. Seek a more comprehensive understanding and provide a higher level of intensity.

What an attractively menacing, youthful lady you are! If you engage in inappropriate speech, I will cleanse your language with a fluid of mine."

I deeply appreciate the incredible growth of your confidence and presence when I engage in conversation with you in such a manner.

I deeply value indulging in the process of consuming your rooster. In addition, I will thoroughly cleanse it by licking.

Please engage in sexual intimacy with me, my partner, and allow me the pleasure of tasting your bodily fluids.

I could spend an extensive amount of time exploring the intimate region between your thighs, engaging in subtle acts of pleasure such as caressing, giving oral stimulation, and savoring the taste of your essence.

I need you. I desire to engage in sexual congress with you. I would like to express my gratitude for the intimate experiences we share. I would appreciate engaging in sexual intercourse with you.

Oh, my dear, that was the most enjoyable intimate experience I have ever encountered. I am greatly indebted to you for that.

Please refrain from being serene within the confines of this room. Instead, endeavor to exemplify behavior that is respectable and be mindful of engaging in inappropriate or vulgar conversations.

Benefits And Distinctions Of Modern Sexual Practices Compared To Conventional Methods

There exists a distinct disparity between tantric sex and conventional sexual intercourse, with individuals often underestimating the profound influence exerted by tantric practices and their transformative potential on one's sexual experiences.

An Alternative Route

Regular sexual activity consists of three distinct phases: preliminary activities, the act of engaging in sexual intercourse, and culminating in the climax or final phase. Upon completion of that task, it signifies its culmination, and typically, one's involvement is concluded. Occasionally, one engages in intimate relations and subsequently returns to their customary routines.

However, tantric sex diverges from conventional practices. Tantric sexual practices do not exhibit any linear progression. It is plausible that one may not experience orgasm until after engaging in both foreplay and intercourse, or perhaps foreplay alone can facilitate reaching that state. The idea behind it isn't to just focus on the orgasm, and don't use the orgasm as the ending point. It dispels that notion and consequently diminishes fixation on it.

The prevailing energies exist in that place.

The energy exhibited during a typical sexual encounter differs. It is a solely carnal encounter, involving the interaction between male and female reproductive organs, wherein the entirety of the experience is centred on physicality. Whether it involves kissing, caressing, grasping, or even engaging in sexual intercourse, the underlying essence is purely physical, lacking substantial mental stimulation. Frequently, individuals may fail to engage in mutual eye contact, and it is imperative to acknowledge that this characteristic distinguishes tantric sex.

The profound bond experienced during tantric intercourse extends beyond the realm of physicality, representing a distinct form of energetic manifestation. This encompasses more than mere sexual energy; rather, individuals endeavor to channel and diffuse this energy from the genitalia throughout their entire being, resulting in various forms of pleasure. The gratification and vitality present are not solely derived from physical movements, but also from the emotional and intellectual state of your partner. It facilitates a heightened emotional connection, rendering it a substantially more intimate endeavor compared to conventional sexual encounters in the majority of instances.

Collaboration "Cooperating in unison "Joint efforts "Collective labor "Mutual participation

The aspect associated with conventional sexual activity typically involves reaching an orgasm as the ultimate objective, aimed at achieving a sense of release and subsequently concluding the act. You are placing a greater emphasis on that rather than simply collaborating and savoring the present moment in each other's company.

An intriguing aspect of tantric sex is that one can achieve orgasm not solely through the act of intercourse itself. Certain individuals experience heightened pleasure and sensory stimulation through the means of massage therapy, gentle sexual stimulation, and even various forms of nipple stimulation, thereby attaining a state of tantric orgasm. The concept revolves around reducing excessive concern regarding orgasms, and instead, directing attention towards the present moment.

It is important to ensure that your breathing aligns with that of your partner, maintaining a harmonious rhythm without any discernible signs of respiratory strain or inconsistency. It is also important to maintain interlocking gazes with each other.

This is a phenomenon that escapes the awareness of a significant portion of individuals when they partake in conventional sexual activity. Whether it be engaging in intimate acts from behind or simply preferring to have the lights dimmed rather than bright, individuals are hesitant to establish direct eye contact with one another. Perhaps it is the susceptibility inherent in this juncture, yet it has the potential to alter one's emotional state. Engaging in tantric intercourse fosters a shift away from individualistic thinking, prompting a more altruistic mindset and facilitating the gradual cultivation of a deep, intimate bond.

Duration

The duration of sexual activity typically varies, and it is customary for individuals to spend no more than an hour engaged in such intimate encounters, unless they deliberately choose to engage in prolonged sessions. Occasionally, the expedited sessions conclude in a mere five minutes, concluding thereafter. However, it should be noted that tantric sex has the potential to endure for an extended duration, often spanning several hours.

This is primarily due to the fact that their motivation is not solely driven by personal pleasure, but rather, they seek to engage in a deep, immersive connection where they can mutually engage in intimate relations. It is worth noting that tantric sex elicits a greater number of orgasms and more intense orgasms compared to conventional sexual activity.

The culmination of the game does not involve the exhaustion of physical energies. Rather, it entails a cyclical progression wherein both individuals derive enjoyment and pleasure from each other, along with the expenditure of pleasure and intensity.

The Emotive

The drawback inherent in conventional sexual activity is its primary emphasis on tactile stimulation, lacking the potential for transcending beyond the physical realm. However, what is intriguing about tantric sex is that, in certain instances, physical contact between the participants may be absent. On occasion, individuals may simply make minimal gestures in that area, while on other occasions, they experience a heightened sequence of pleasurable sensations.

It additionally generates waves of orgasmic stimulation. This is because tantric sexual practices entail experiencing a profound and enchanting wave of pleasure that extends beyond the surface level, encompassing the transformative power of orgasm. It is truly remarkable how transformative this experience can be, as it evokes profound sensations of pleasure and ardency.

Tantric sexuality does not necessarily entail extensive physical contact, nor does it necessitate the inclusion of intense discomfort or any elements of this nature. Alternatively, it could manifest as a sequence of distinct and intensely pleasurable climaxes.

The remarkable aspect of tantric sex lies in its incorporation of a profound and captivating manifestation of energy between partners, which serves to cultivate and expand one's capacity for sensual gratification.

The Most Potent Energy

Certain individuals may hold the belief that tantric sex might not possess the utmost level of potency, yet it undeniably possesses substantial strength. The reason for this is rooted in the inherent nature of human connection facilitated by energy, whereas physical intimacy, while involving touch, may not always encompass the same level of profound connection. Tantric sexual practices can be compared to the yogic techniques of transcending the physical realm, similar to how yoga surpasses the typical physical exertion of a conventional gym workout. Both options are commendable, however, it should be noted that seeking a profound physical and emotional bond with one's partner often manifests through the practice of tantric sex, as opposed to engaging in conventional sexual encounters.

Tantric sexuality encompasses the entire physical being, permeating it much like a sponge absorbing and subsequently emanating the entirety of that vital energy.

Tantric sexual practices present a means by which one may actualize the essence of their being. This is precisely why some individuals contend that tantric sex constitutes the most potent expression of physical intimacy, as it encompasses the spiritual dimension inherent in the act of lovemaking. It constitutes a type of intimacy that is highly legitimate and encompasses a multitude of principles that are undeniably valid and deserving of recognition.

Due to that singular factor, Tantric sex emerges as the preferred form of sexual engagement. It facilitates a profound and meaningful bond with the individual you hold dear.

Through the practice of tantric sex, individuals have the opportunity to forge a profound connection with the divine, immersing themselves in the sublime magnificence of this unique experience. It affords a heightened spiritual and gratifying intimacy, permitting one to engage with the transcendent. Tantric sexuality serves as a remarkable means to foster a profound sense of intimacy between you and your partner.

Enhances Interpersonal Bonds

Individuals often fail to recognize that engaging in sexual activity does not inherently imbue significance or emotional resonance on the part of one's partner. Occasionally, engaging in sexual activity occurs solely for the purpose of gratification or seeking pleasure, without truly experiencing the profound and enjoyable connection that accompanies an intimate relationship with one's partner.

Indeed, while engaging in sexual activities may be enjoyable and foster intimate bonds for certain individuals, a potential concern lies in the tendency for such encounters to give rise to a somewhat superficial connection within the relationship. Certain individuals engage in sexual activity solely to maintain their relationship, whereas tantric sex is not driven by such motives.

Not all sexual encounters are pursued with the intention of cultivating a meaningful bond. At times, this behavior is pursued solely to achieve orgasm without any further intention or purpose. But tantric sex lets you foster a better, deeper connection with your partner, and allows you to have empowered sexuality via arousal and stimulating the senses. One begins to witness a resurgence of the profound sensual aspects of intimacy, wherein individuals acknowledges that it fosters a deeper, purposeful connection with their significant other.

Numerous individuals hold great admiration for this particular form of intimacy as it fosters a deeper and more profound connection with another individual. Individuals desire to demonstrate affection and devotion to their significant others, and tantra, in particular, offers a unique opportunity to deeply experience passion and invigorate intimate connections.

You strive to introduce novel ideas and tantric sex offers you the opportunity to accomplish this goal.

Romantic gestures are not extinct; rather, individuals often become preoccupied by monotonous patterns. Tantra is a way for you to keep sex alive and well in your life. And you don't even need to believe in antra to do it. If you are interested in experiencing the various positions and exploring the pleasurable aspects of physical intimacy, you can readily engage in it through sexual activity.

Many individuals are unaware of the shifts occurring in their relationships, and may not even acknowledge the importance of their partners' presence. However, by engaging in tantric sex, individuals can cultivate a more profound and meaningful bond with their beloved, as well as establish a stronger and more dependable relationship with themselves and their partner.

Is Tantric Sex Better?

It is important to note that it is not suggested that one completely abstain from engaging in sexual activity on a regular basis. One is encouraged to engage in sexual activities in a manner that aligns with their personal preferences. However, it is important to acknowledge that the practice of tantric sex encompasses the stimulation of the entire body and necessitates embracing a state of vulnerability and well-being. For a significant number of individuals, the experience of tantric sexual practices is contingent upon the depth of the bond and affection one shares with their intimate partner. For those who have harbored curiosity regarding tantric sexual practices, engaging in such activities can be a truly beneficial experience.

However, the characteristic of tantric sex lies in its prolonged duration, as it is devoid of any defined objective or endpoint. If you desire to engage in conventional sexual activity with your partner, you may proceed, although it is crucial to acknowledge that it may not foster a profound emotional bond.

Can tantric sexual practices contribute to the preservation and enhancement of intimate partnerships? However, it is essential to acknowledge that sexual intimacy alone cannot resolve all issues within a relationship. Therefore, in the case of a failing relationship, it would be prudent to explore alternative methods and strategies in order to maximize the satisfaction derived from your sexual partnership. For many, tantric sex builds it all, and makes it so that you're able to build and foster that connection with people that you love. The significance of the person whom you hold dear is of great importance, which is why numerous individuals derive pleasure from engaging in tantric practices. This is because the significance lies not only in the physical act, but also in the emotional connection and love shared between individuals.

Having comprehended this, you shall realize how tantra enhances the holistic well-being, whereas conventional sexual activity primarily focuses on the physical aspect. Both experiences are highly enjoyable, however, if one desires to cultivate a more profound and meaningful bond with their beloved, tantra provides the optimal means to achieve this objective.

This is why tantra is highly regarded as it facilitates the cultivation of affection and comprehension between individuals in an intimate relationship. It can enhance your physical well-being, promote overall wellness, and contribute to increased levels of personal happiness as well.

So, which is best? The correct response is tantra; however, it is crucial to grasp the distinctions as well. Both of them possess advantages and disadvantages, and you will come to realize that, through every moment and experience shared with your partner, there are numerous benefits to be gained and many that you should certainly strive to embrace.

What Is The Appropriate Age To Introduce Comprehensive Sexual Education To Your Child?

It is imperative that children are provided with appropriate sexual education at an appropriate age in order to prevent them from deviating from the right path. As per the insights of industry professionals, it is deemed crucial to impart age-appropriate and tactful sexual education to children.

It is possible to commence at the age of four or five years. Familiarize young children with their genitalia at a young age. It is imperative that comprehensive information regarding intimate anatomical regions, including their respective nomenclature, be provided. Both appropriate physical contact and inappropriate physical contact should also be addressed.

Children aged eight or above demonstrate an increasing capacity to comprehend and assimilate information through the medium of television and the internet. In the present era of advanced technology, it is incumbent upon parents to diligently oversee the sexual conduct of their children and furnish them with relevant knowledge.

As per Sychar's findings, it has been observed that children frequently inquire about the manner of their birth. Regrettably, a significant portion of parents tend to evade providing a response to this inquiry. Therefore, in response to this inquiry, it can be affirmed that the woman's uterus, encompassing a sac within it, serves as the dwelling place for the fetus wherein it undergoes a developmental period of approximately 9 months before ultimately being delivered into the world.

By the time a child reaches the age of 10, parents must exercise heightened caution. The occurrences of sexual assault that are reported in the daily newspaper ought to be deliberated upon with the family during the morning meal or afternoon tea. This will help ensure that even the youngest ones remain vigilant upon hearing it.

Engage in communication with individuals who are older than 15 years

During adolescence, individuals exhibit heightened intellectual capacity, demonstrated by higher cognitive abilities by the age of 15. During this stage of their development, they also cultivate their comprehension. In such scenarios, it is crucial to comprehend the cognitive processes of the children, alongside imparting knowledge on sexually transmitted infections such as HIV and AIDS. Nevertheless, parents should consider certain factors when introducing their children to sex education, beginning with determining the appropriate age to commence.

Dr. Elizabeth Oyenusi, a consultant pediatric endocrinologist, expressed the viewpoint that parents should initiate sexual education for their children at the earliest opportunity. She elaborated that the optimal timeframe for this would be between two to three years, taking into consideration that it aligns with the stage when children generally commence venturing outside, be it for educational or other purposes.

Therefore, it is important for parents to instruct children on the identification of their anatomical features and delineate the boundaries of appropriateness. During this time, parents should also provide children with clear instructions regarding appropriate boundaries for physical contact, emphasizing that if any unwelcome encounters occur, they must promptly notify their parents."

Given the potential for exposure to potentially harmful content on television and other media platforms, it had become imperative to provide them with education at such a young age. Children should be introduced to these fundamental concepts at a young age, preferably around the age of eight. As responsible parents, it is important for us to provide clear and explicit guidance in these matters as they mature. This phenomenon is particularly relevant during that stage in a girl's life when she starts to experience breast development, which may generate interest among individuals, particularly among men, given the notion of attractiveness.

Regardless of the child's gender, once they reach the age of eight, it is essential for parents to have a conversation with them concerning sexuality. It is imperative that during this discussion, parents refrain from using colloquial terms or visual aids, particularly considering the exposure that children receive from various media sources such as television and the internet.

A young lady is prepared for such instruction when her bodily development commences or when she turns eight years old."

Inquired about the most effective method for initiating the process of educating children on matters related to human sexuality. There is no definitive guideline concerning the approach, as there are children who inquire and others who do not pose questions.

Parents have a responsibility to respond to inquiries posed by their children, while also taking the initiative to introduce specific terminology to those who do not ask, thus obviating the necessity for the use of informal aliases or nicknames. Parents may also inquire about their existing knowledge to determine the next steps to be taken."

Considering that children have commitments outside of their residences, particularly those who have returned to educational institutions, and given the presence of opinions asserting the unique responsibilities of parents and teachers in child development.

As parents, you possess a paramount responsibility as you hold the primary position in understanding your child, whereas the role of teachers serves as a supplementary asset.

Parents need to first equip their children with basic knowledge, and whatever the teachers do will only complement what they have been taught already.

It would be judicious to initiate a discussion with them about sexually transmitted diseases and infections, given that they could potentially arise from engaging in sexual activity."

Additionally, Dr. Rotimi Adesanya, a consultant pediatrician, emphasized that the long-term consequences of not providing early sexual education to children could prove exceedingly burdensome, as they are prone to acquiring misinformation from unreliable sources.

He articulated, "The insinuation is that upon their departure from parental guidance, such as for educational pursuits, their susceptibility to misinformation increases as they have not received proper instruction regarding moral discernment."

Sex education encompasses more than simply instructing children about sex and advocating for abstinence; it also involves imparting knowledge about the anatomy and physiological functions of the reproductive system in a systematic manner.

For instance, consider a child who has not received early guidance from their parents regarding the negative perception of homosexuality or lesbianism. In such a case, the child might lack an understanding that inappropriate touching by an individual of the same sex or opposite sex is morally unacceptable.

However, if the parents have instilled the belief that individuals of the same gender should not form intimate relationships, this information would be assimilated and retained within their cognitive faculties. Therefore, if anyone were to execute such an action, their options would be limited to either fleeing or alerting authorities. Hence, it is imperative for parents to impart such knowledge within the confines of their own households, in order to safeguard against the acquisition of erroneous information from external sources.

It is not unusual for a young female to be misled into believing that engaging in sexual activity could alleviate the discomfort associated with menstruation. Given her vulnerable nature, she may inadvertently become susceptible to exploitation, as she believes it might alleviate her suffering.

However, had she received proper instruction regarding the ineffectiveness of sex in alleviating menstrual discomfort, she would not be susceptible to deception and would exercise caution towards any man making such claims.

Typically, young females, around 10 or 11 years of age, experience the onset of menstruation, marking the commencement of adolescence. This is the opportune time for mothers to initiate discussions regarding maturity, imparting knowledge about the physical changes that adolescents can anticipate, such as breast development and the onset of menstruation, which may occur unexpectedly.

At this stage, it is advisable for parents to instruct their children to keep a safe distance from any situation that may prompt them to unzip or discard their trousers.

Regarding the appropriate age at which children should be educated about sex, considering the current prevalence of information and communication technology (ICT) where information cannot easily be concealed, it may be imperative for parents to introduce sex education to their children as soon as they acquire the ability to read. Nevertheless, it is crucial for the content of the sex education to be tailored and presented in a manner that aligns with the child's level of comprehension.

It is imperative to streamline the information and explicitly specify the areas of the anatomy that are to be avoided. There exists a musical composition that elucidates the notion that certain anatomical regions ought not to be physically contacted. Parents can extend their efforts to the extent of engaging in singing with their children and discerning those particular areas.

It is imperative to provide children with education that encompasses foundational concepts, such as the inherent distinction between boys and girls as ordained by a higher power. As simple as it is, while in preschool, girls should be told that there should be no hugging.

Nobody should hug them. If anyone persists, they ought to inform these individuals that their mother typically embraces them, which should suffice. It is imperative to instruct children on the importance of promptly signaling or vocally alerting others in case of any suspicious circumstances.

It is imperative to instruct them on anatomical structures and their respective functions, elucidating the potential risks and reasons behind refraining from engaging in any form of sexual activity. It is imperative that parents refrain from utilizing the term 'things' when referring to genitalia, and instead employ the appropriate anatomical terminology for these organs.

Please inform them that this is a domain that ought not to be explored until the bonds of matrimony have been sealed. They should be educated on the inappropriate nature of males touching a female's chest or back pockets."

As children progress in age, particularly during their mid-primary years and as they approach entering secondary school, it becomes imperative to enhance their education regarding appropriate boundaries. It is crucial to educate young males about refraining from touching the chest or private areas of females, and to educate young females about refraining from touching or striking boys in the genital region.

Commencing at an early age with age-appropriate education about sexuality is highly advisable.

The inquisitiveness surrounding sexuality is an inherent development that stems from acquiring knowledge about the human anatomy.

Comprehensive sexual education aids adolescents in gaining a thorough understanding of human anatomy, fostering a positive body image and promoting self-confidence. Adolescents exhibit curiosity towards pregnancy and infants, rather than delving into the intricacies of sexual mechanics.

Furthermore, engaging in conversations about sexuality is an integral aspect of fostering open and honest dialogue with one's child. Effective, sincere, and transparent communication between parents and children holds immense significance, especially as your child enters adolescence.

When fostering an atmosphere of open communication, adolescents become more inclined to engage in meaningful conversations with their parents regarding a wide range of adolescent challenges including but not limited to anxiety, sadness, interpersonal relationships, substance abuse, and sexual matters.

Chapter One

The Warm-up

Prior to delving into proper communication with unfamiliar acquaintances, it is imperative that we consider the following:

Your warm-up

Your methodology

Furthermore, the events preceding the collaboration...

We will take into account this individual's preliminary actions. In order to avoid a distant collaboration, it is necessary to adopt a cordial approach. When initiating contact with someone for the first time, it is crucial to convey "Friend Signals." Upon our initial encounter with someone, our cerebral faculties must hastily discern whether this individual should be categorized as an ally or a foe. In order to acknowledge the aforementioned two entities, the subsequent points serve as a couple of directives to be observed:

Adversary Signals:

Crossed arms

Lack of direct visual contact
Secret hands
Companion Signals:
Establishing a channel for non-verbal communication; ensuring an unobstructed path with no hindrances in the middle.
Maintaining direct eye contact upon approaching
Evident hands poised for a handshake.
Whenever you encounter another person, it is imperative to employ accompanying cues when approaching them. You will also enhance your level of concentration by smiling at them.

The Opener
Given your approach of displaying friendly and welcoming nonverbal cues, what would be your verbal communication with the individual? The mere thought of pick-ups and opening lines tends to induce high levels of anxiety in individuals, yet I assure you there is no need for such apprehension. The significance of the initial line is not as profound as it may seem.

Conversations that are truly exceptional and yield great results are also the most effortless. Can you confirm whether or not you are adequately prepared for the situation?

The best opening line is... 'Hello, how are you?' Simple right? It is simple and successful to open a line. Therefore, refrain from driving yourself to madness by devising something astute or ingenious. Please greet the individual by saying, "Hello, how are you?"

The Shake

Subsequently, or upon first encountering, extend your hand in a firm and respectable manner for a handshake. Regardless, consider a situation in which you are not an influential figure. Considering the highly unpleasant situation, I strongly advocate for you to proceed and extend your hand to the other individual, at the very least. Why? Given the substantial importance of handshakes. Upon the moment of contact between your skin and another individual's skin, your body releases substances that facilitate the process of grasping or holding onto objects. Should you desire to further enhance your mastery of the artful practice of the ideal handshake, we invite you to peruse the instructional video provided below. Allow us to impart upon you a few fundamental principles to bear in mind for your future handshaking endeavors: ensure your hands remain devoid of moisture and execute your handshake with a resolute grip.

The Intro

Currently, it is the opportune moment to introduce yourself. Once you initiate the conversation with a polite greeting such as "Hello, how are you?", it is essential to commence cultivating compatibility. The approach to achieve this entails commencing with your personal identity and the manner in which you have manifested yourself. Additionally, should it be possible for you, kindly return it to them. An example would be, "To illustrate, I might introduce myself by stating, 'Greetings, my name is Vanessa.'" This marks my inaugural attendance to this gathering. How about yourself?" Then their response would enable them to anticipate the unforeseen. You are presently engaged in a discourse, thereby transcending your previous status as mere observers.

One final suggestion I would like to offer is to incorporate the use of food and beverages as an initial conversational tool, whenever feasible. Engaging in conversation with the person next to you is facilitated by choosing to sit at the bar, as it requires the least amount of effort. Approaching the buffet line in order to engage in conversation is quite mundane. As an entire collective, we engage in the consumption of food and beverages, making it a straightforward point of entry.

Allow me to offer you a piece of advice that may not have been imparted to you by your mother: Engage in social interactions with unfamiliar individuals and observe how effortlessly you can engage in conversation with anyone. Meeting strangers tends to evoke apprehension in most individuals, second only to public speaking. Thankfully, this encounter does not have to be as disconcerting as one might initially anticipate. The following ten straightforward suggestions will help you engage in comfortable communication with an unfamiliar individual.

Following That, The Matter Of 'Where' And 'When' Arises.

The location and timing of discussing matters of sexual intimacy with your partner hold significant importance, potentially outweighing the actual content of the conversation. Here, planning is everything

It is important to allocate dedicated time to discuss matters pertaining to your sexual relationship.

The Setting (WHERE)

While the presence of a nearby couple listening in on your conversation with your partner may not be a concern or bother you, it is important to consider that a crowded restaurant may not be the most appropriate setting for engaging in such a deeply personal discussion.

It would be advantageous to engage in the discussion within a secluded setting, such as during an intimate meal prepared at home, a leisurely stroll, or while comfortably situated on the couch/in the bedroom. Any environment chosen should provide privacy, comfort, and minimal distractions. In a scenario where you are both in isolation, you will have the liberty to engage in unrestricted communication, free from concerns about potential eavesdropping.

When considering the location aspect:

Set time and communicate

Select a mutually convenient time and engage in prior communication with your partner to discuss these matters, refraining from catching them off guard with impromptu conversations pertaining to topics such as orgasms, G-spot stimulation, penile rings, and similar subjects.

In a more formal context, it might be phrased as follows: In the course of an ordinary discussion, inform your partner in a diplomatic manner that you wish to engage in a conversation concerning your intimate relations. It is advisable to articulate your specific topics of interest in order to foster a more effective dialogue.

The appropriate timing for the conversation should be:

A time that accommodates the availability of both individuals

Select a time in which neither party is experiencing excessive fatigue; designate a timeframe when both you and your partner are in a state of relaxation, potentially during a leisurely Sunday morning.

When both individuals are in a positive disposition, it becomes readily apparent to discern the emotional state of one's partner. Engaging in communication with your partner during periods of anger, sadness, or irritation may inadvertently obfuscate the intended message, hindering the ability to convey thoughts and feelings in a transparent and concise manner.

Please be aware that your partner may not be receptive to

If you experience a sense of discomfort when broaching the subject, it is highly likely that your partner experiences similar sentiments as well.

After broaching the topic of engaging in a discourse surrounding intimacy, it is crucial to maintain composure and refrain from taking umbrage should your partner display initial hesitance. Despite potential initial resistance from your partner, if the relationship holds significance for both individuals, they will inherently desire to engage in discussions aimed at enhancing the overall relationship.

In the event that your partner may feel hesitant or reserved, it is advisable to provide them with reassurance by emphasizing the significance of engaging in open discussions about sexual matters. Furthermore, expressing your willingness to approach these discussions with an open-minded attitude can be highly beneficial.

"Once the WHERE aspect is adequately prepared, redirect your attention towards the what:

The Content (The WHAT)

It is imperative to have a clear understanding of the topics you wish to discuss with your partner at all times. It is imperative not to merely inform your partner of their shortcomings without offering any further guidance or support.

If the subject pertains to the attainment of sexual climax, feel free to mention it. If it pertains to aspects that cause a decrease in interest or enthusiasm, kindly express those concerns while maintaining a tactful approach. To facilitate the process of determining one's speech content, it is recommended to adhere to the subsequent guidelines:

Examine your intimate relationship with your partner carefully. Consider occasions when the sexual experience was profoundly satisfying, as well as those instances where it did not meet your expectations.

Please document the specific elements that you found enjoyable and those that were not favorable.

Reflect upon your desires and contemplate the various experiences you would be inclined to pursue with your significant other, subsequently documenting them for reference.

Please document any inquiries or concerns related to sexual matters.

Now you have the option to select any of the aforementioned topics that you wish to address at a specific time or, alternatively, engage in a comprehensive discussion in a single session—feel free to even consider seeking the assistance of a sex therapist!

Understanding the appropriate occasions to refrain from discussing matters pertaining to sexuality carries equal significance to comprehending the appropriate moments and suitable language to engage in such conversations.

Instances Where Having a Discussion Is Inadvisable

As previously stated, certain situations that may appear opportune for discussing matters related to sexual concerns can have adverse effects on the interpersonal dynamics within your relationship.

"Refrain from discussing sexual matters in situations like:

During the intense exchange of diverging opinions

Even if you deem a matter of a sexual nature as significant to an intense discourse, refrain from introducing it into the course of such a discussion. It is difficult to predict your partner's reaction, and it is highly likely that your partner will not receive it favorably.

In a state of intense displeasure, one's verbal expressions may become less guarded, resulting in unintentional miscommunication. In moments of anger, when emotions are heightened, we occasionally exhibit impulsive behavior or utter impulsive remarks. Once we regain composure, rational thinking resumes.

Abstain from discussing matters of a sexual nature amidst a contentious disagreement. Take a moment to allow your partner to relax and compose themselves, and then initiate a discussion on the matter.

During sex

Broaching the topic of sexual matters during moments of intimacy appears to be a prudent suggestion. The reason behind this is that when engaging in such behavior, one tends to become distracted from the task at hand, namely, the focus on one's partner.

If you have been in a long-term relationship and unexpectedly propose that your partner engage in toe-sucking during a sexual encounter, it can profoundly surprise and dishearten your partner, ultimately leading to a loss of intimacy and connection. Conversely, if it is a matter that has already been deliberated, proceedings would proceed smoothly, resulting in immense satisfaction for both you and your feet.

It is imperative to clarify that this does not imply refraining from communicating your desires, instructing your partner on where to touch you, or indicating what actions to take. It simply indicates that astonishing your partner, particularly with a divergence from the norm, is not regarded as the pinnacle of excellence. Provide your partner with advance notice.

Over text/phone call

Discussing matters of a sexual nature via telecommunications, particularly through text messaging, may appear significantly more comfortable and devoid of awkwardness. However, the potential for misinterpretation and miscommunication in phone or text interactions should not be underestimated.

To begin with, your partner lacks the ability to perceive your nonverbal cues and vocal intonation. Consider the hypothetical scenario wherein your romantic partner communicates via written correspondence their disdain for the manner in which you express pleasure during intimate moments. Contrast this with the scenario where your partner respectfully approaches you and expresses that at times your vocalizations might divert his/her focus during intimate moments.

Regardless of the medium through which you present it, whether it be text or phone communication, it is undeniable that the impact of a conversation conducted in person is unrivaled.

Through the involvement of an intermediary

Discussing one's sexual experiences with the company of a third individual is generally ill-advised. The sole circumstance in which it can be deemed acceptable is when the third party involved possesses professional qualifications, such as that of a sex therapist.

Sex is a private and personal experience shared exclusively between individuals in a committed relationship; effective communication is crucial for its successful realization. It is worth considering that your acquaintances and loved ones may have some suggestions, however, it is important to bear in mind that irrespective of their opinions, ultimately, only you and your significant other possess the true understanding of what is most suitable for you both.

Discussing matters related to sexuality is not as intricate as it is frequently perceived to be. When a couple maintains effective channels of communication, discussing topics related to sexual intimacy can be a pleasurable experience. There are numerous conversations that are significantly more uncomfortable than discussing sex, particularly when you are in a dedicated partnership.

Allow us to address the diverse and fundamental aspects pertaining to sexuality that warrant discussion in order to enhance both the quality of your relationship and the intimacy within your sexual encounters.

Protocol For Engaging In Conversations Regarding Puberty With Your Daughter

When engaging in a conversation with your daughter regarding the topic of puberty, it is essential to bear in mind that your objective is to adequately equip her with the necessary knowledge and understanding in anticipation of what lies ahead. This is also an opportune moment to provide her with reassurance regarding the normalcy of the changes she will encounter. At present, your daughter may experience a sense of insecurity regarding her physical appearance. She may undergo abrupt increases in breast size and hip prominence, experience a growth in height, encounter the emergence of acne on her previously unblemished face, as well as manifest fluctuations in mood. For a young individual, these transformations can be intimidating and perplexing. As a parent, it is incumbent upon you to provide reassurance to her that these physiological changes precipitated by the onset of puberty are acceptable and indeed within the realm of normalcy.

A selection of the physiological transformations that can be anticipated during adolescence:

Girls:

It is probable that their height will increase.

• The individual may begin experiencing the development of acne

• The mammary glands are undergoing maturation and will experience growth in size.

• The hips and legs will adopt a more curvaceous shape.

• The onset of pubic and axillary hair growth will commence.

• There will be an overall darkening of hair growth on the body, potentially resulting in increased thickness as well.

• will commence menstruation

• May undergo fluctuations in mood

Boys:

• The occurrence of pimples and acne is possible. • Pimples and acne may manifest. • Pimples and acne have the potential to emerge. • Pimples and acne have the propensity to form.

• is anticipated to experience a period of rapid and significant growth

• The vocal pitch becomes lower.

• The prominence of the Adam's apple becomes apparent.

• The onset of facial hair growth commences • The emergence of facial hair becomes apparent • The development of facial hair initiates

• The growth of pubic hair and underarm hair will commence.

• The size of the penis and testicles increases

• Experience nocturnal emissions • Encounter episodes of spontaneous sexual arousal during sleep • Engage in involuntary sexual experiences during dream states

- Individuals may undergo shifts in mood.

It would be beneficial to communicate to your daughter regarding the transformations affecting not just females but also males. This will assist her in navigating interactions with male peers within her age group as well as individuals beyond her age.

137

It is crucial to underscore that each individual girl and boy possesses distinct attributes, and the process of development during puberty may vary among individuals. It can present challenges for an adolescent girl to navigate social interactions when she finds herself as the sole participant who has commenced the process of puberty. Alternatively, in a contrasting fashion, the outcome is equivalent for an individual who has not yet undergone puberty while their peers have commenced encountering the aforementioned transformations. Repeatedly emphasize to her that each of her acquaintances will inevitably experience puberty and that it is entirely normal to experience it earlier or later than others.

CHAPTER THREE

The Guidelines for Engaging in Electronic Sexual Messaging:

1. Get (and give) assent/consent.

Similar to the essential consideration of consent in any form of sexual engagement, it is equally crucial to obtain consent before engaging in sexting with someone.

It might be considered atypical if they are in a meeting, especially if they are sharing their screen and forgot to disable notifications. Alternatively, they could be engaging in leisure activities."

This holds additional importance particularly if you are sharing an intimate self-portrait. Regard the act of seeking consent as an effective means of encouraging your partner.

If your partner involved in sexting is making you uncomfortable (or if you have received an important phone call in the midst of sexting), please be aware that you have the option to withdraw consent at any time.

2. Please refrain from disseminating any explicit or compromising visual content of your partner at any given time.

Please refrain from disclosing or sharing any communications received from your partner to third parties. This encompasses not only photographs and recordings, but also encompasses any desires or aspirations shared by your partner. It is imperative that you exercise caution when mentioning to others that you and your partner engage in sexting, unless you have previously confirmed with your partner that they are comfortable with such discussions.

3. Safeguard your protection.

In the event that you intend to transmit visual or auditory media, it is imperative to exercise caution and only engage in intimate interactions with a trusted individual. Just because someone appears attractive or you are involved in intimate relations with them does not justify confiding your explicit photographs with them. Engaging in a romantic relationship or sexual encounter does not necessarily imply a willingness to send such images. It is crucial to be mindful of the legal statutes concerning sexting in your jurisdiction, particularly if you are underage.

It is advised to exercise caution when transmitting unambiguous facial codes or symbols in most cases. Attempt capturing images by angling the camera downwards from your face, allowing your partner to appreciate the allure of your lips while avoiding concerns about excessive visibility. Many individuals usually opt to incorporate counterfeit tattoos into their photographs as an additional measure to ensure personal safety, making it more challenging for others to identify their actual appearance.

When storing visually appealing images on your mobile device, consider utilizing a distinct application to avoid the inadvertent exposure or transmission of intimate photographs from your photo application.

4. Show appreciation and energy.

Sexting often induces feelings of anxiety or helplessness in individuals, particularly when explicit images are involved. It is advisable to provide ample positive reinforcement within the conversation to foster a sense of confidence and well-being regarding the content being shared.

Due to the fact that your associate is unable to perceive your tone of voice or observe your body language, you have the ability to make a significant effort by employing emojis, exclamation marks, and adjectives. The heart and kiss emoticon serve as a suitable point of initiation, and the heart-eye and slobbering emoticon are excellent options to express your partner's capacity to arouse you through their words or pictures.

It is also opportune to express to your partner, 'You are arousing intense desire within me at this moment,' or 'Your allure is awe-inspiring.' Please refer to the examples provided below for further illustrations of expressing gratitude through verbal and pictorial means.

5. Endeavor to refrain from casting judgment on your partner's aspirations.

Sexting can serve as an effective means for individuals or their partners to establish a heightened sense of security when divulging concealed fantasies or desires that have not been previously disclosed. Endeavor to avoid inducing feelings of regret or dissatisfaction upon others by passing judgment on them or engaging in actions that result in them experiencing genuine remorse for their choices.

If the assumption they are alluding to via explicit communication is genuinely detrimental to your state of mind, we recommend redirecting the conversation away from that particular topic or circumstance. For example, in the scenario where your associate has mentioned the idea of restraining you but it does not align with your preferences, an appropriate response could be: "Given that I prefer to use my hands to explore your body, I kindly request that you release me so that I may assume a position where I can be on top."

6. Take things gradually.

Sexting as a form of foreplay holds comparable significance to conventional foreplay.

Often, we mistakenly transmit an excessive amount of intimate content prematurely. This is because the allure of sexting predominantly lies in the intensification of sensuality and anticipation."

Certainly, when engaging in sexting, one has the ability to prolong and stimulate their partner to a greater extent due to the lack of risk in getting overly excited or progressing too rapidly, as one would in a face-to-face interaction. Commence by illustrating the surroundings, the mindset of both yourself and your associate, the attire chosen by each party, and similar details. Consider potentially stimulating your partner by transmitting a suggestive message, followed by instructing them to contemplate it while you attend the gym. Promise to share a perspiration-inducing photograph upon your return.

7. Acquire a high level of proficiency in the language they wish to learn.

Does your associate appreciate it when you address them as the term 'child young lady'? Alternatively, do they prefer being referred to as a prostitute? What term for their intimate regions elicits the most intense sensation? Here are all the factors to consider before engaging in sexting with someone else (and it is always advisable to revisit these points with your current partner).

If you are uncomfortable engaging in a prelude conversation before sexting, you may attempt incorporating this approach into your sexting dialogues. For example, do you experience sexual arousal when I address you as 'Daddy'? It is readily apparent that when making such a inquiry in this particular circumstance or manner, your significant other may feel a heightened inclination to acquiesce, albeit with certain expectations of avoiding offense. Therefore, it is imperative to bear this in mind.

8. Ensure that your messages of a sexual nature are clear and unambiguous.

Currently, it is not opportune to distance oneself or feel ashamed about one's imperfections. The degree to which you clearly articulate your requirements and preferred methods of communication will greatly enhance clarity and effectiveness in working with your associate. Efficiently convey your preferences, desires, and expectations in a coherent manner, regarding your enjoyment and the treatment you desire, along with expressing your appreciation for the actions you expect from the other person in that given moment."

If you have reservations about your writing abilities, it would be advisable to contemplate the five senses when crafting your explicit messages, taking into account elements specific to your partner, such as their physical attributes, sexual preferences, or even the environment in which they reside.

9. Endeavor to refrain from perspiring over the visuals.

Engaging in explicit messaging can bring complete enjoyment without exchanging symbolic gestures, and it is crucial to never transmit any content that makes you uncomfortable, particularly if your partner is pressuring you to do so.

To impress your sexting partner, amplify the disturbance. Instead of submitting a reflection of your unclothed physique, please provide a photograph that captures nearby items from a lower perspective or a video showcasing a gradual tactile motion along your body. Occasionally, donning scant attire such as a sheer blouse or limited clothing can generate more allure than being completely unclothed. Alternatively: From time to time, adorning oneself with minimalistic garments, such as a translucent top or skimpy clothing, can evoke a heightened sense of sensuality compared to complete nudity. Furthermore, there is no need to become overly concerned about capturing a photograph that is deemed visually appealing for Instagram. One aspect that contributes to the appeal of exchanging provocative images is their authenticity and rawness. Additionally, the realization that your accomplice captured a photograph exclusively for you can be greatly exhilarating to certain individuals.

10. Attain equity: The feeling of security afforded by an electronic interface can transform sexting into a remarkable instrument for you and your partner to delve deeper into each other's sexual

preferences and potential desires. Please do not hesitate to inquire for further clarification on urgent matters. When you arrive this evening, what attire would be appropriate for me to wear at the entrance to greet you? I would be greatly aroused if you were to perform oral sex on me from behind, or alternatively, if you were to pleasure my testicles orally, it would drive me to a state of intense desire.

11. Diligent adherence to a set of principles yields favorable outcomes. In acquiring any new skill, there is an inherent expectation to assimilate information. Ensuring certainty, along with the provision of assertive statements from your accomplice, is of utmost importance. Please be reminded that your sexting partner is not expecting award-winning writing or photographs. A component of what stimulates them is the recognition of the identity concealed by the telephone screen.

CHAPTER 2

The psychological underpinnings of vulgar language and its enhancement of sexual gratification.

Similar to the case of sexual role-playing or setting the mood with lighting, engaging in explicit language is a matter that strongly relies on individual preferences. For certain individuals, it is an innate aptitude. For some individuals, it requires effort and dedication. For some individuals, it is a profoundly displeasing form of cognitive exercises, akin to reciting your timetables while being penetrated. It facilitates cerebral engagement while disconnecting from one's physical embodiment.

That being stated, based on recent research findings, it has been revealed that the use of explicit language is consistently regarded as one of the most popular sexual inclinations or preferences shared by individuals of both genders worldwide. Therefore, for individuals who appreciate a measure of verbal interaction alongside the physicality inherent in a sexual encounter, it is important to recognize that you are not alone in this preference. For individuals who have yet to engage in the practice of enhancing intimate relations through the use of provocative language, it may be advisable to contemplate the potential merits of doing so.

Undoubtedly, it can be challenging to comprehend the rationale behind engaging in explicit language while already partaking in intimate activities. However, it appears that a significant portion of sexual arousal is derived from cognitive processes within our brains. These neural circuits are activated in novel and enhanced manners when we partake in the practice of explicit verbal communication during intimate encounters.

However, it has been widely established that auditory stimulation during sexual activity is arousing. Expressing the same idea in a formal tone: "Vocalization, from both the participant and the observer, can play a significant role in many of our sexual fantasies, and auditory cues associated with sexuality can likewise stimulate those cognitive processes."

Furthermore, engaging in sexual intercourse can alleviate self-consciousness, resulting in individuals feeling more comfortable discussing fantasies, intense desires, or unconventional preferences while in the midst of the act. To clarify, if you are inclined to explore BDSM, role play, or other intimate aspects of kink, engaging in explicit language could serve as a valuable avenue for exploration prior to delving into more physically involved practices.

Regarding the topic of role play: In the event that you and a partner are involved in enacting character roles or engaging in a dominant-submissive dynamic, the use of explicit language serves as an additional means of solidifying that narrative. Indeed, in numerous instances of role-playing scenarios, it is the most inherent method of immersing oneself in the persona.

Furthermore, research has indicated that engaging in explicit conversations outside of the intimate space can greatly enhance the sexual experiences of a couple. If you introduce dirty talk in the un-self-conscious, candid space that is the bedroom, then you're far more likely to feel comfortable broaching the matter in other walks of life—which can be a particularly fiery turn-on for most couples and a way of instigating sex without being, well, unsubtle.

I had never anticipated developing an interest in explicit conversations prior to experiencing it firsthand. I hold a great appreciation for accuracy, and I would reserve the term "daddy" solely for individuals who truly fulfill that role. Nonetheless, on the initial occasion, an individual committed the unimaginable act of vocalizing suggestive language to me during a sexual encounter (via erotic expressions, rather than innocuous inquiries or my customary banter), and curiously enough, I experienced arousal. I was pondering the psychological aspects underlying explicit language and the arousal it elicits in individuals to vocalize things in the intimate setting (or any location of sexual activity) that they typically would not express.

One potential explanation for the apparent enjoyment people derive from engaging in explicit discussions is rooted in the notion that sexual activity serves as a mechanism for relieving stress. Consequently, individuals engaging in such conversations may experience decreased self-awareness, thereby being more inclined to openly express their actual thoughts, actions, and emotions. Based on research conducted by the National Center for Biotechnology Information in 2005, it has been observed that experiencing an orgasm stimulates the release of oxytocin, a compound known for its stress-reducing properties. Reducing your stress levels implies a decrease in inhibitions and an increased likelihood of expressing your true thoughts and desires, even if you typically refrain from doing so in your daily life. Perhaps you have something of a suggestive nature to express about your partner's physique, but you may feel hesitant to articulate such thoughts due to various personal reasons; nevertheless, those sentiments inadvertently escape at the peak of the situation. If one harbors particularly explicit thoughts, it is more probable for them to be expressed as one reaches climax.

The usage of explicit language stimulates our neural activity, which is in fact a significant source of sexual arousal. You may be familiar with the expression "thinking with your lower head" (essentially referring to the penis), however, it is important to note that your upper head—the brain—is actively involved in this process. Sexual stimulation is not solely reliant on reproductive organs, as other factors also play a significant role in this process, although it is worth noting that sexual organs hold their own importance. The impact of brain function on sexual pleasure may elucidate the reasons behind a diminished desire for sexual activity in instances of unhappiness or heightened stress levels.

Based on a study published in Hormone Research in 2005, it was determined that the preoptic area and the suprachiasmatic nucleus of the hypothalamus are accountable for the experiencing of sexual pleasure. Engaging in explicit discourse arouses the interests of both parties, inducing a state of sexual readiness in individuals. According to the publication Cosmopolitan, engaging in verbal expressions or soft vocalizations during sexual activity elicits a neurochemical response that enhances arousal in both individuals involved. If you experience heightened sexual arousal in response to verbal communication, there may exist a plausible explanation for this phenomenon.

Certain individuals derive pleasure from the experience of engaging in submissive discourse, particularly when they occupy significant positions of authority in their everyday existence. The use of explicit language elicits a response in the amygdala, which serves as the brain's fear center and regulates arousal and gratification. According to the American Dating Society, individuals experience similar emotions that generate a sense of fulfillment through assuming responsibility, and these very sentiments also result in individuals feeling stimulated by yielding to authority.

Similarly, dirty talk makes the dirty-talker appear confident, so it can be a role reversal if one person is more confident in their everyday lives. Not all individuals are aroused by explicit language that evokes a sense of submission, therefore it is important to

engage in a conversation with your
partner prior to attempting it.

www.ingramcontent.com/pod-product-compliance
Lightning Source LLC
Chambersburg PA
CBHW051734020426
42333CB00014B/1311